Dedicated to our son;
siblings of disabled children
are exceptionally special.

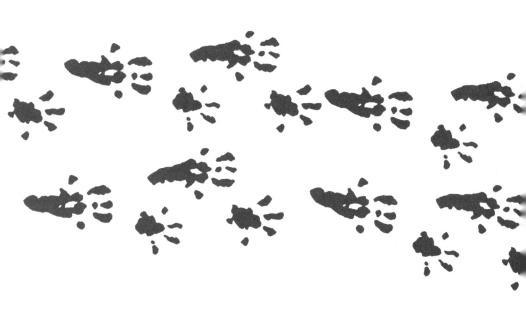

www.2petrats.com

Written and produced by

Nathalie Wendling and Thomas Glatzmayer

Graphics by JG Productions, Oakville, Ontario, Canada

Photography by Photoluxstudio, Ottawa, Ontario, Canada

Inquiries about this book should be addressed to:
John William Glatzmayer, Manotick, Ontario, Canada

Melanie & Tommy
have two pet rats
and one syndrome

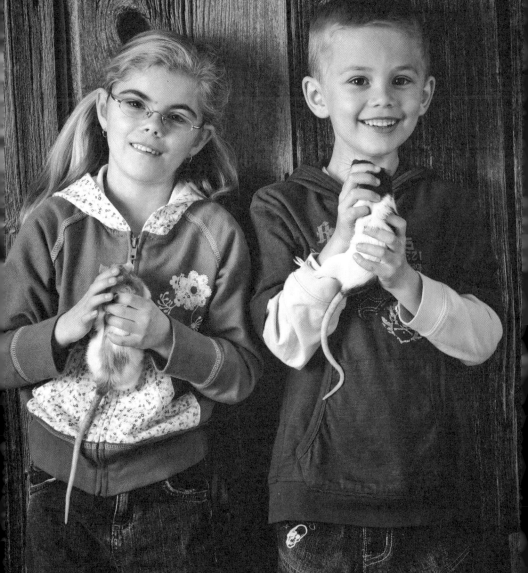

By Nathalie Wendling and Thomas Glatzmayer

Photographs by Photoluxstudio

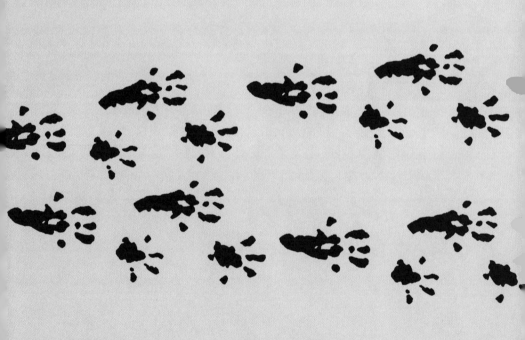

Down syndrome …

Autism…

Tourette's syndrome…

It's not like a mosquito bite.

My sister was born with

Cornelia de Lange Syndrome…

and it won't go away

overnight.

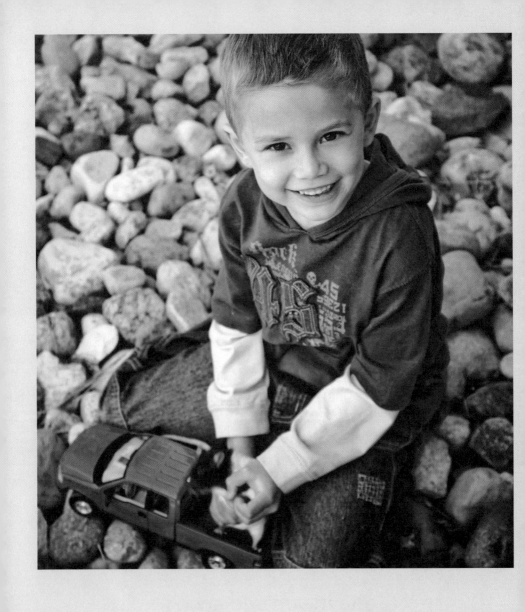

My name is Tommy.

I am six years old.

I like vehicles, villains and victory.

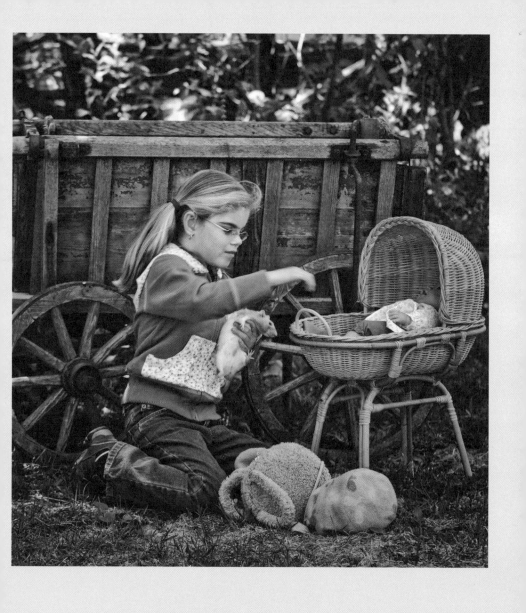

My sister's name is Melanie.

She is nine years old.

She likes bags, bubbles and her baby.

Chapter 1

We live on a farm in the cold country of Canada.

Our parents are busy raising lambs and llamas.

Every day we have specific chores.

On Mondays, we go to the grocery store.

Today, there are three items on the list:
eggs
bacon
and
mocha java.

I bought my car at an auction.

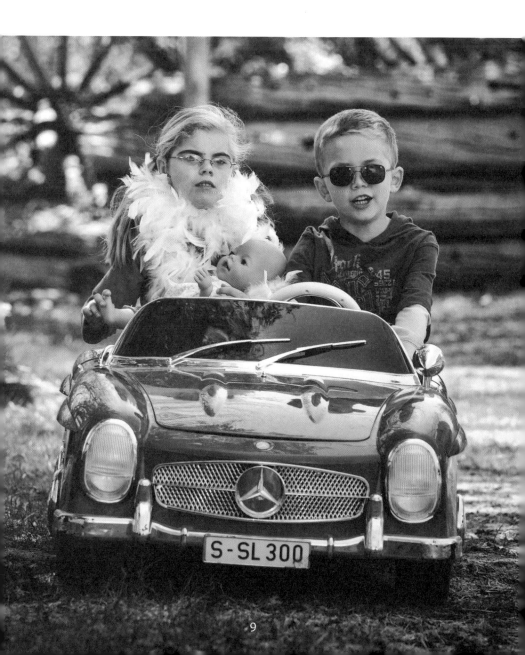

Stop!

Oops! I almost forgot...

It's time for Melanie's medication.

She has an ear infection.

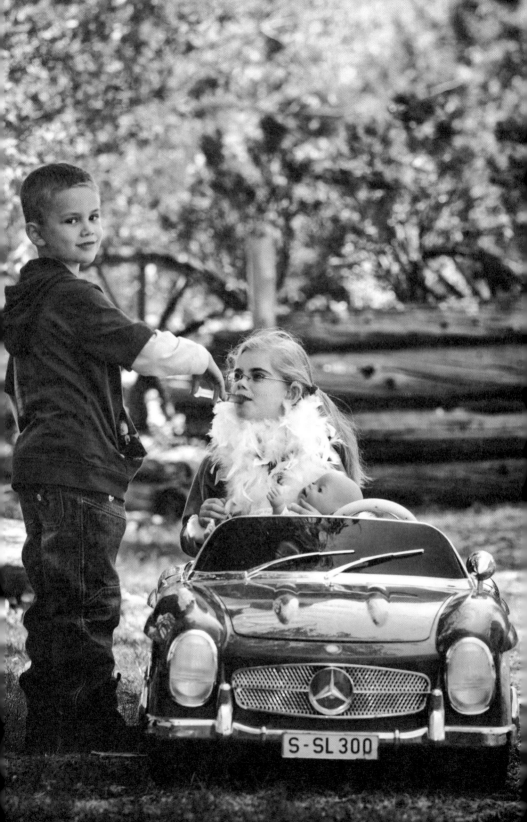

The road was really bumpy.

I was driving too fast!

Look out, a hole!

Oh no! We lost control.

Smash!

Crash

Bash

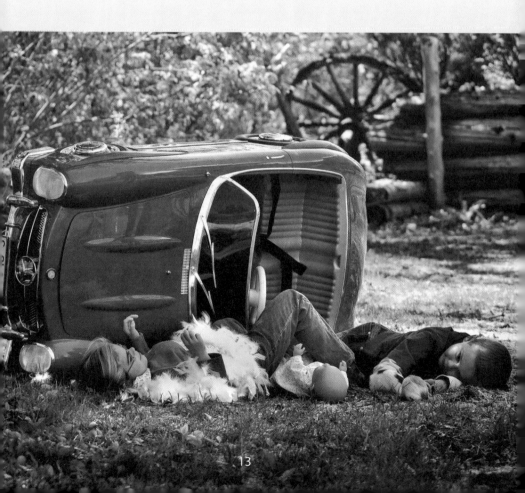

The
rats
went
for
help!

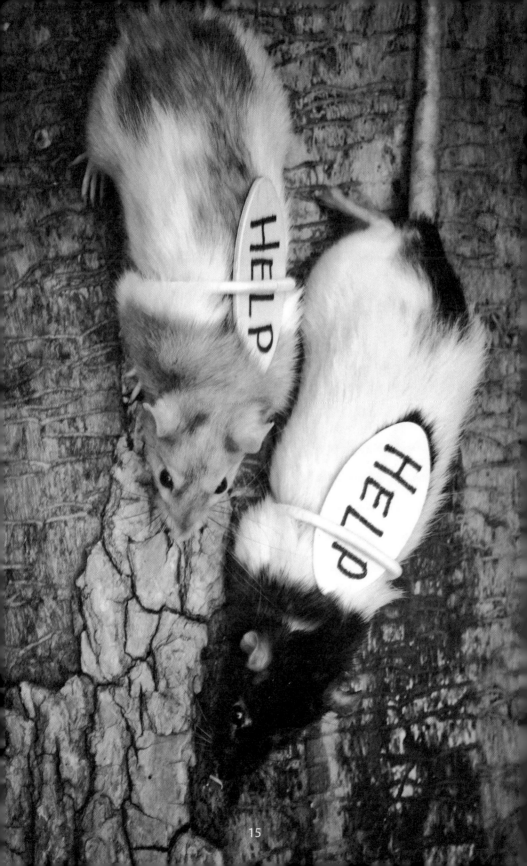

Emergency and rescue vehicles from all

around the world quickly responded.

Police cars, ambulances, fire trucks,

tractors, tanks, tow trucks and

bulldozers.

I even heard a helicopter.

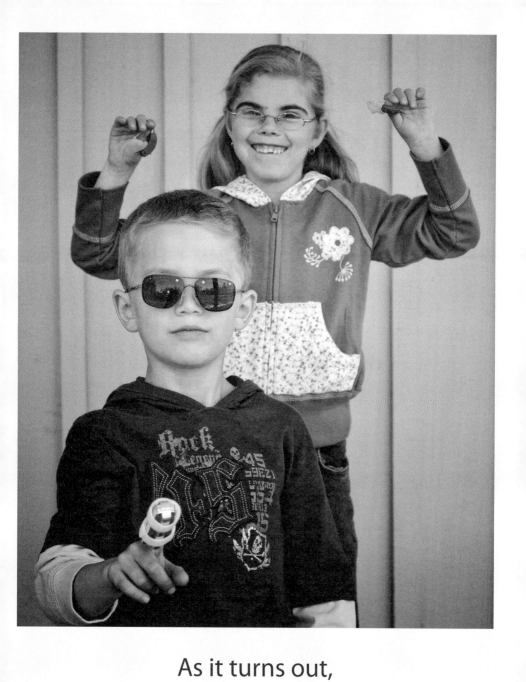

As it turns out,

Melanie's hearing aids needed new batteries

and I broke my finger.

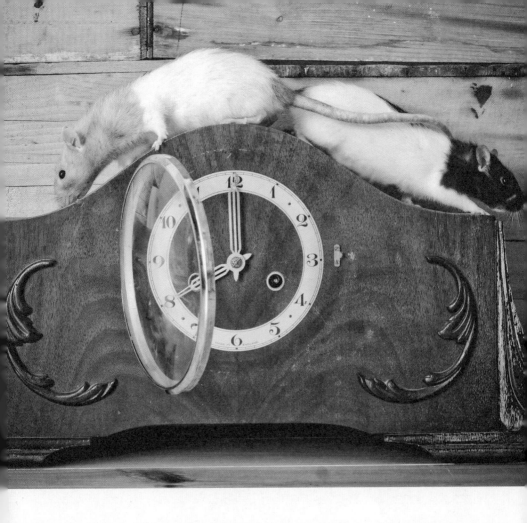

Goodnight... rats

Squeak... squeak

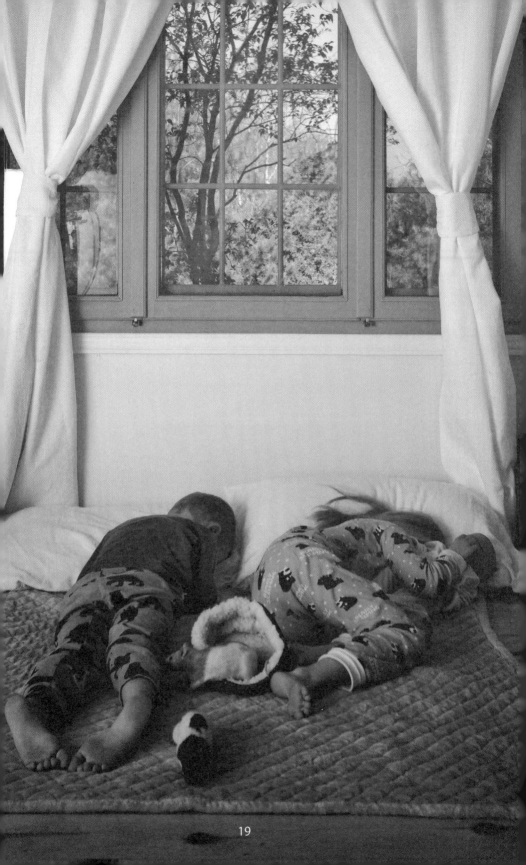

Chapter 2

On Tuesdays we do laundry.

Today, we are on alert!

I am standing on guard.

Billy, the neighbourhood bully,

was somewhere in our backyard.

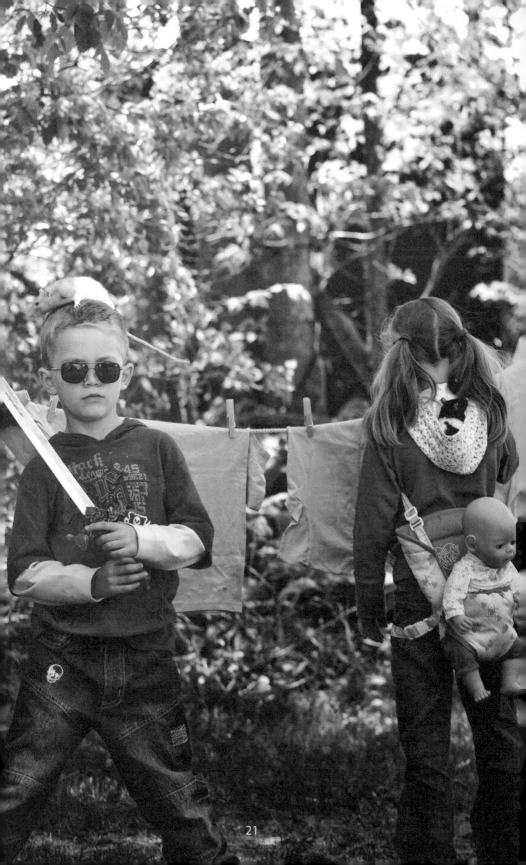

Sometimes,

the rats and I teach

Melanie how to speak.

We make her repeat, repeat, repeat,

repeat, repeat,

and repeat.

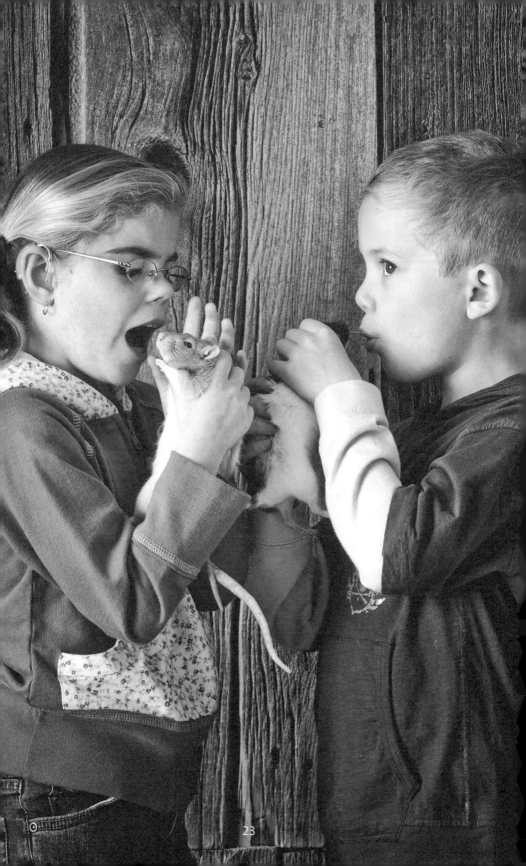

Watch out!

A gust of wind blew the laundry

around,

and around, and around...

We got so dizzy.

Boom!

We both fell down.

Ouch!

Billy!

What are you doing?

Our hands

Oh no!

Our feet!

Stop... Billy!

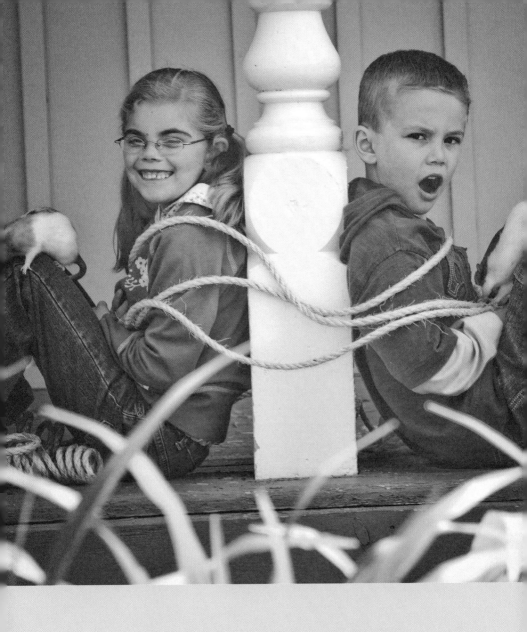

What a bully!

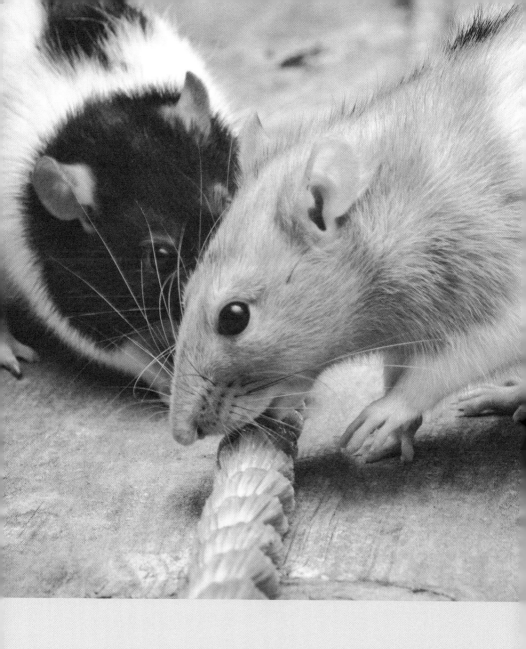

The rats frantically chewed the rope and set us free!

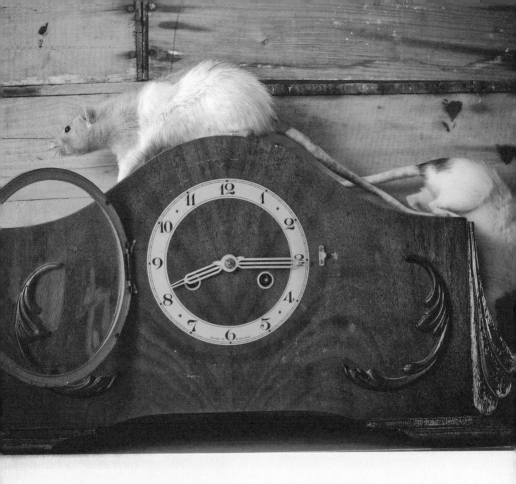

Goodnight... rats

Squeak... squeak

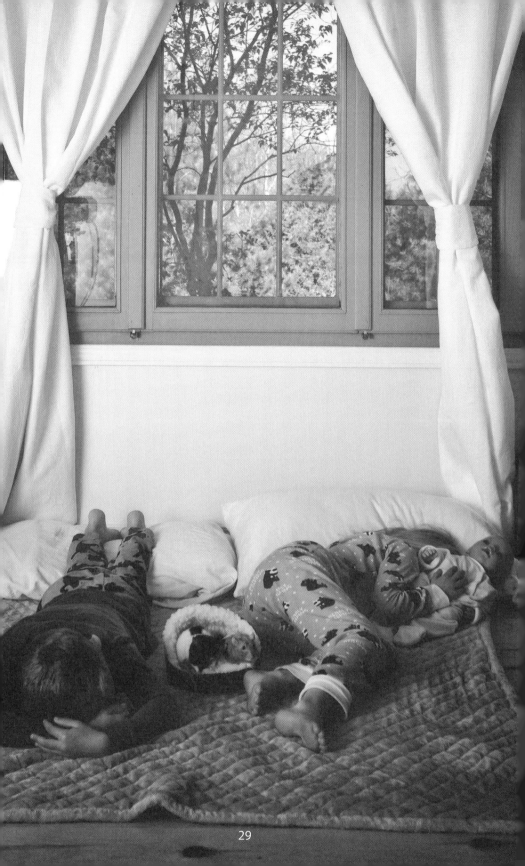

Chapter 3

On Wednesdays, Thursdays, Fridays and
Saturdays, we have more chores.
Chores, chores, chores...

On Sundays, we have NO CHORES.
We play all day!

The day started like any other Sunday;
I got dressed,
then
I helped Melanie get dressed.

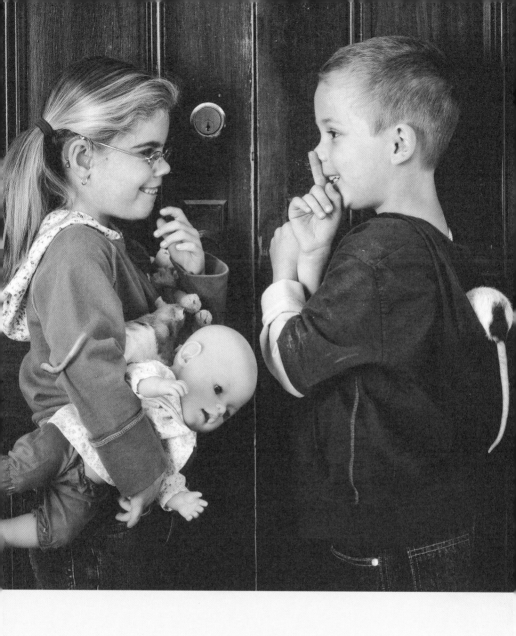

I said Shhh...

Melanie said, Shhhh.

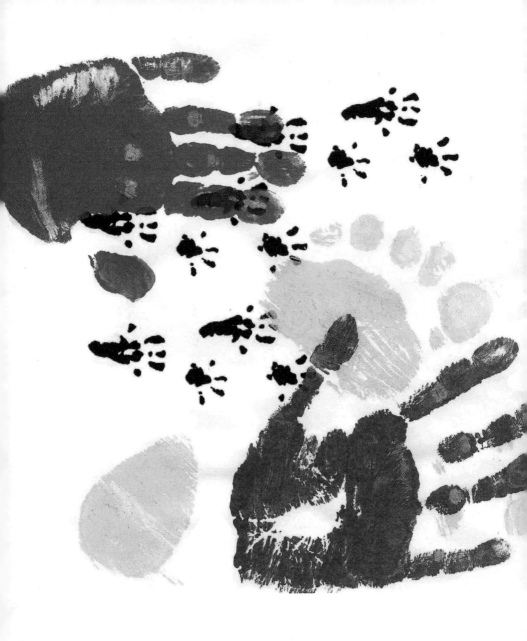

We did some painting!

The rats did some painting!

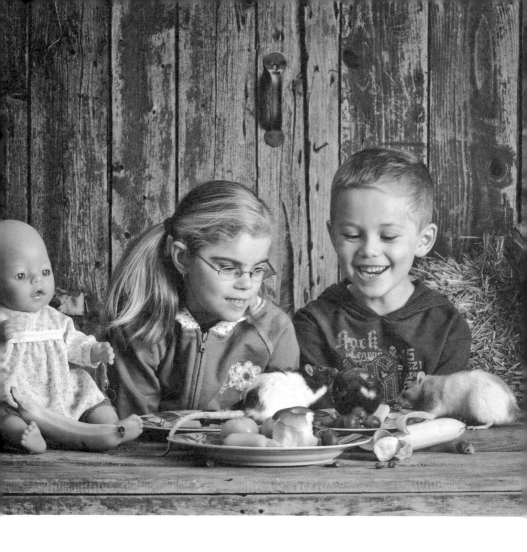

We had a snack.

The rats had a snack.

We were lying in the sun.

The rats were lying in the sun.

Then it happened!

Be careful!

A new litter... four, five, six... done.

By the end, Melanie's rat had

4 daughters and 2 sons.

Wow!

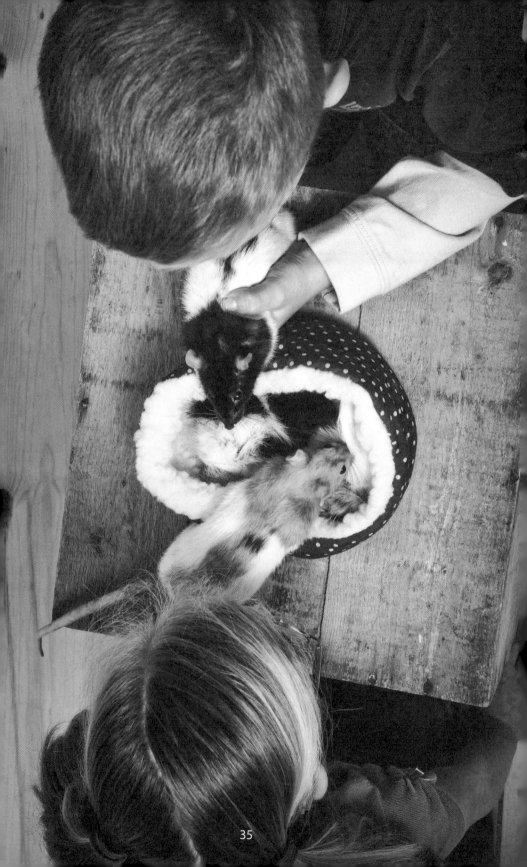

When I grow up, I'll be bigger and stronger.

Melanie will be stronger but always smaller.

Maybe, I'll be a demolition derby driver.

Maybe, Melanie will be a bag designer.

Maybe, maybe not…

Maybe, we will live on the farm together.

Maybe, we will have two houses beside each other.

Maybe, Melanie will marry Billy and have a baby.

Maybe, maybe not…

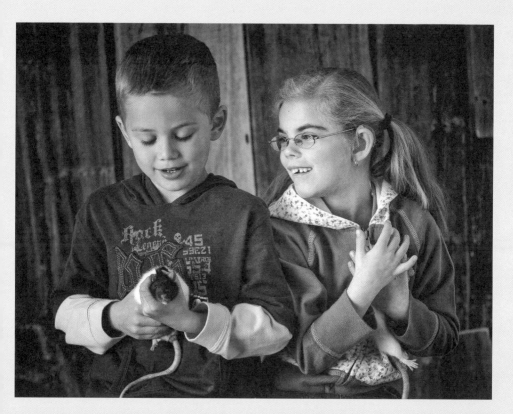

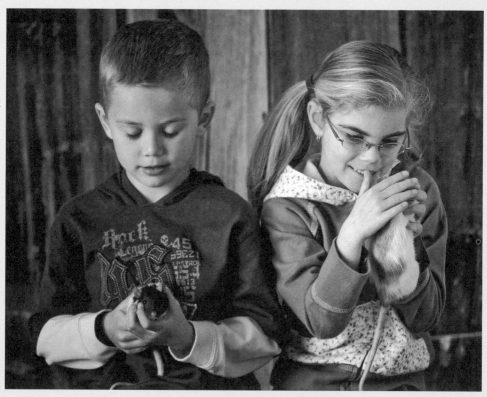

But some things are for sure…

Melanie has a syndrome.

We have so much fun together.

We will be friends forever.

We will have pet rats,

one after another

forever and ever!

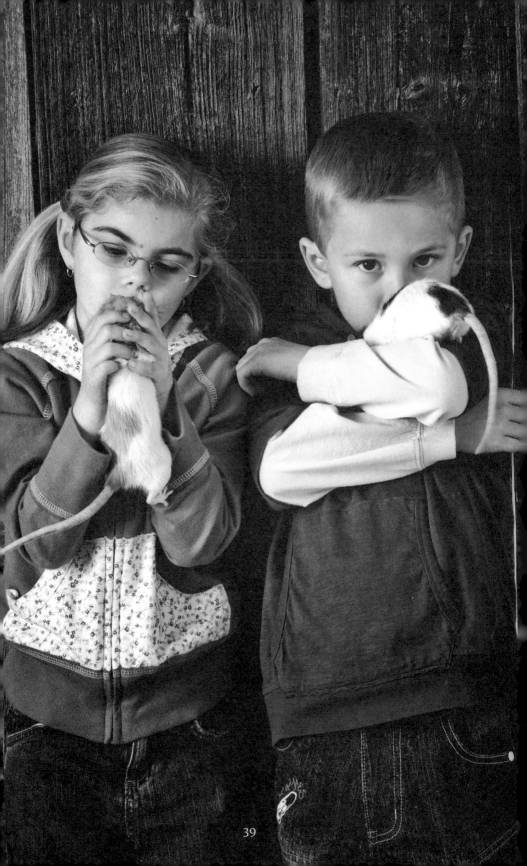

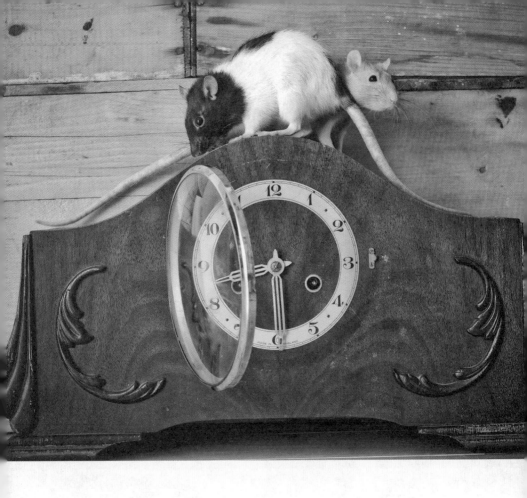

Goodnight... rats

squeak...squeak...squeak...squeak...squeak...

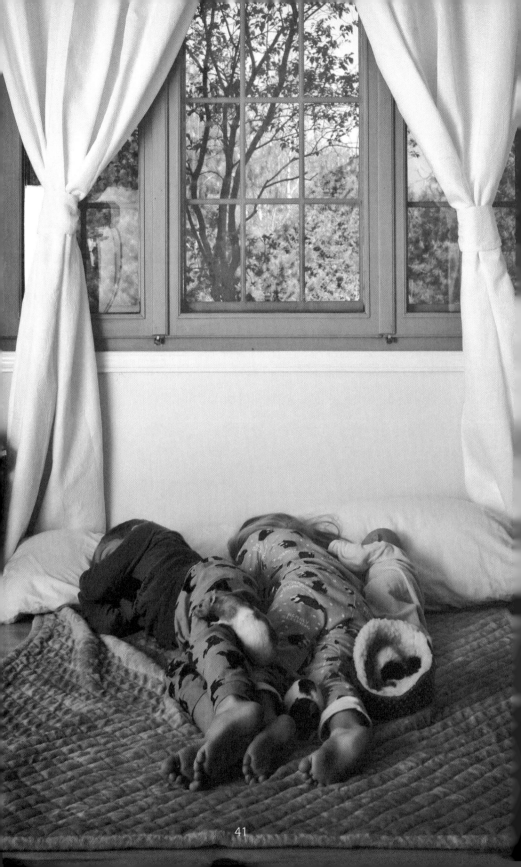

Questions and Answers

What is a syndrome?

You can't catch Cornelia de Lange Syndrome.
It is not contagious.

Melanie was born with it.

Our bodies are made up of skin, blood and chromosomes.
Most of us have 46 chromosomes.

Melanie also has 46 but one of her chromosomes changed
before she was born.

People with Down Syndrome are born with an extra
chromosome, so they have 47.

No one knows for sure what causes Autism or Tourette's syndrome.

Do pet rats bite?

Domesticated rats make great
pets because they never bite.

If you have food on your fingers,
they might be tempted.

Always wash your hands before
holding a pet rat.

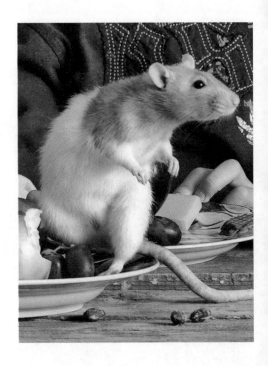

How is Melanie affected by this syndrome?

Syndromes affect people in many different ways.

For Melanie, learning new skills are difficult and take more time.

It took Melanie 5 years to learn how to chew her food.

It took Melanie 9 years to learn how to jump with two feet.

It took Melanie 6 years to say twenty words.

Basic skills like walking, talking and eating are challenging.

Imagine harder skills like reading, writing, skating, cooking, sewing, and driving. They could take years and years of practice.

What do pet rats eat?

Pet rats eat fruit, vegetables, pasta and grains.

We never give our pet rats any meat or sweets.

Their favourite foods are bananas, popcorn and lettuce.

How long do pet rats live?

Pet rats live between 2 and 4 years.

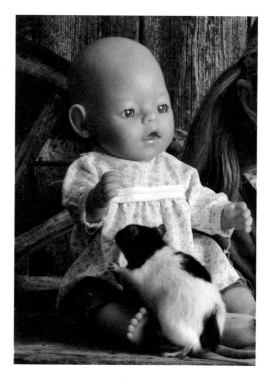

I know staring is rude but I can't stop?

Yes, staring is rude.

But, if you are going to stare at someone for a long time;

wave, smile, say hi,
then smile again!

If the person can't speak, they are usually accompanied

by someone who can.

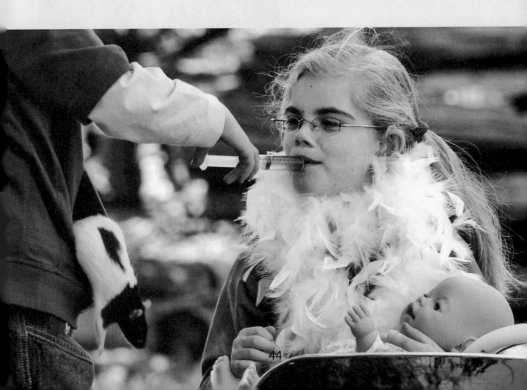

Smile... smile... smile...

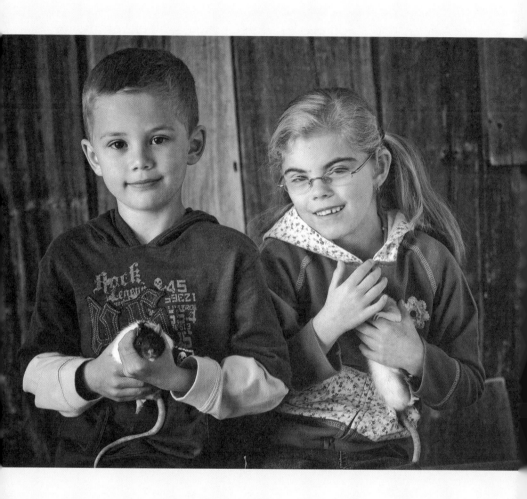

Smiling is not rude!

Cornelia de Lange syndrome (CdLS) is named after Dr. Cornelia de Lange, who first described this syndrome in 1933.

Diagnosis can be made on the basis of clinical observations. The most frequently observed facial characteristics include:

- synophrys (thin eyebrows which frequently meet at the midline)
- long eyelashes
- short up-turned nose
- thin, down-turned lips
- low set ears

Other characteristics often associated with this syndrome include:
- low birth weight
- delayed growth and small stature
- microcephaly (small head size)
- hirutism (excessive body hair)
- gastroesophageal reflux
- seizures and/or heart defects
- cleft palate
- bowel abnormalities
- feeding difficulties
- limb abnormalities - missing limbs or portions (usually fingers)
- absent or delayed speech and hearing abnormalities
- vision problems
- developmental delays
- small hands and small feet
- partial joining of second and third toes
- incurved fifth finger
- 60% – 70% display some degree of autism spectrum disorder.

The estimated birth prevalence is approximately 1:10,000.

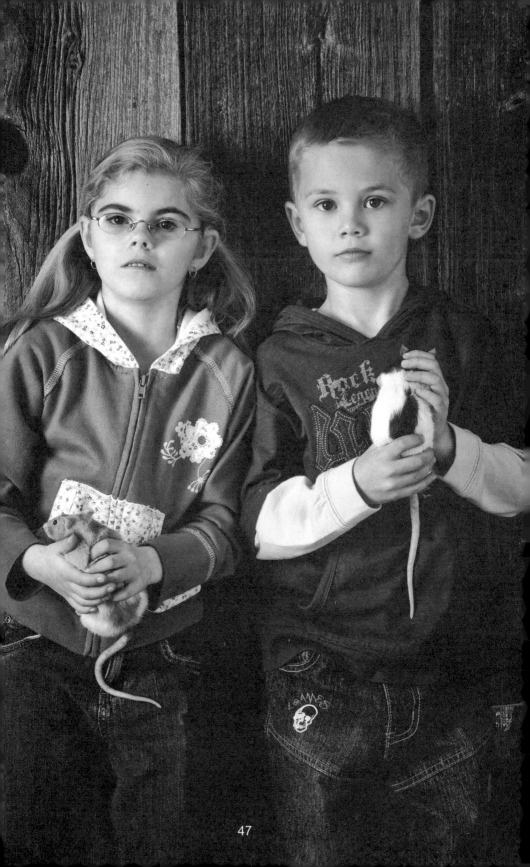

The end.

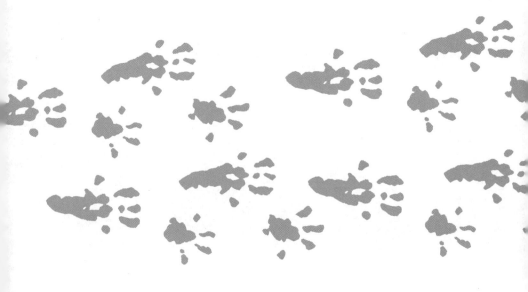

Squeak!